ALLEGRA'S
HOPE

By Samantha Freber

Published by Orange Hat Publishing 2019

ISBN 978-1-64538-064-1

www.orangehatpublishing.com

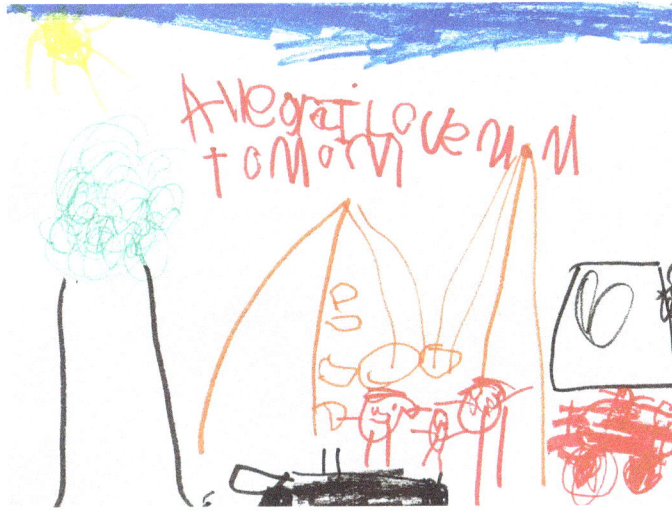

Dedicated with lots of love and heartfelt gratitude...

To our super supportive, generous, dedicated and loving families, friends, Allegra's CF Posse at AFCH, the CF Foundation, and the numerous people we have met along the way.

It takes a village!

XOXOXOXO

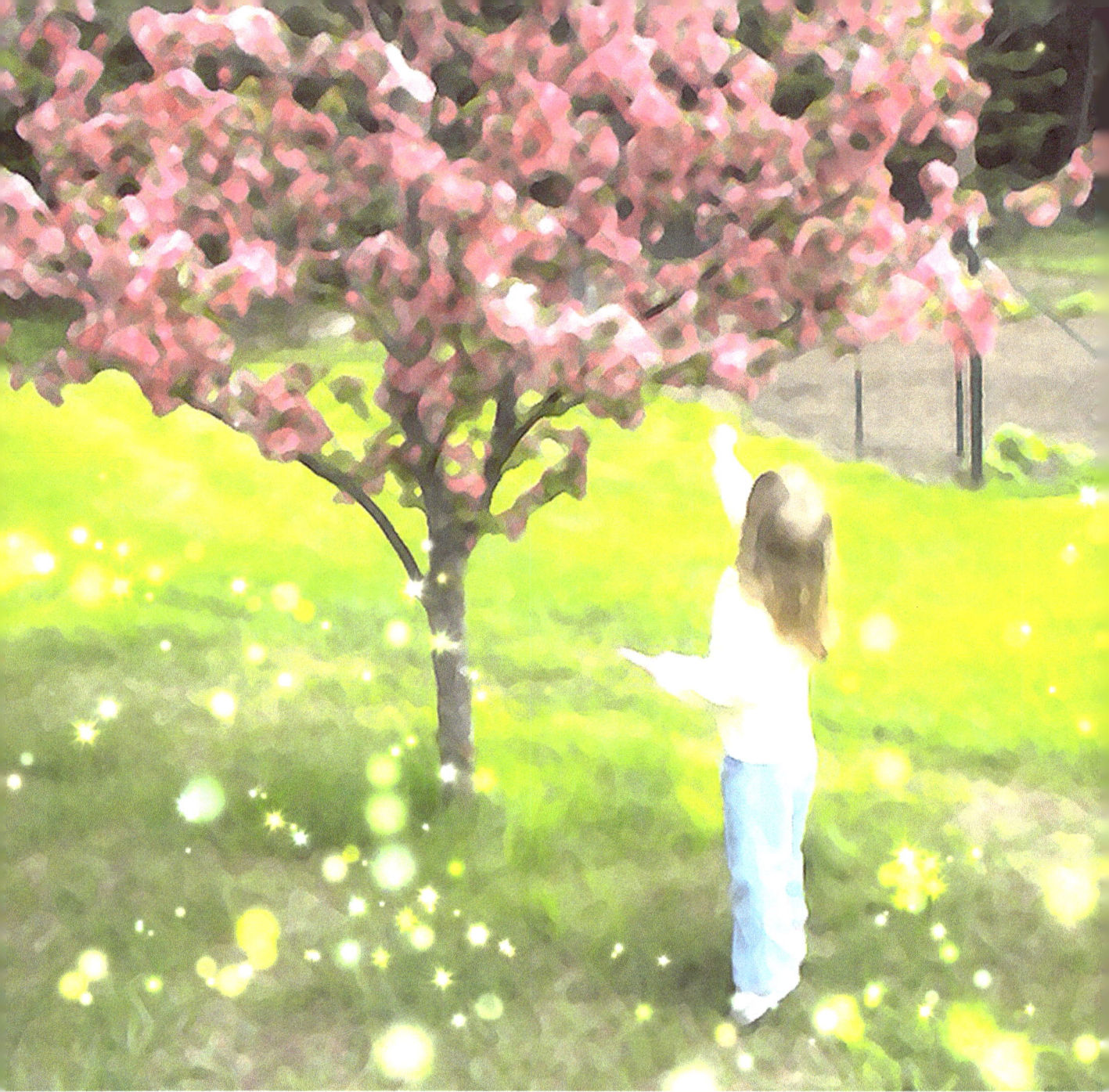

What do you do when you have 65 roses?
Oops, silly me, I mean Cystic Fibrosis?

I bet you'd be surprised to learn
There is less reason to have concern.

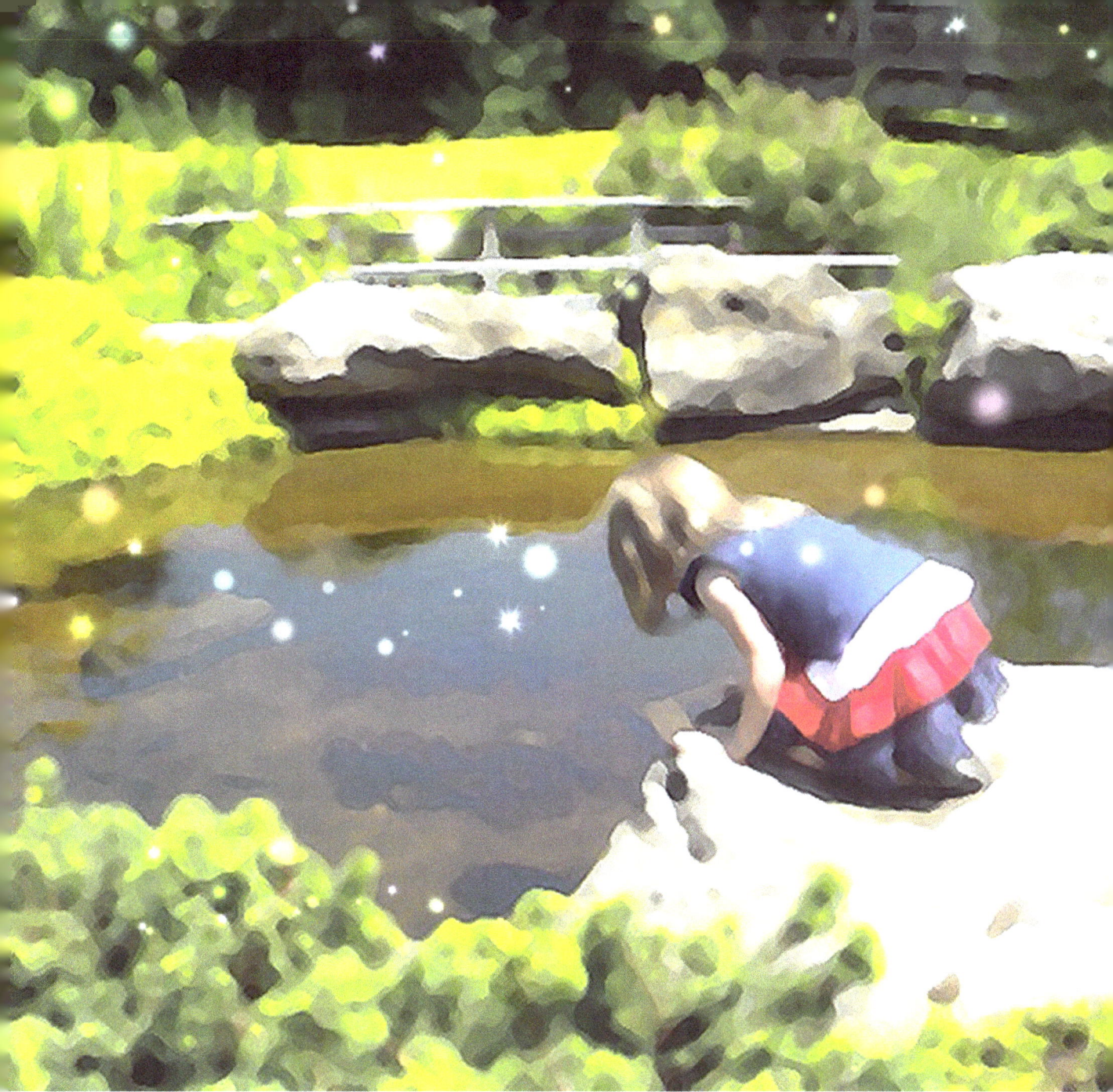

Medical experts have been working hard,
To improve our lives in this regard.

The search for a cure is always in mind.
I have great hope that this they will find.

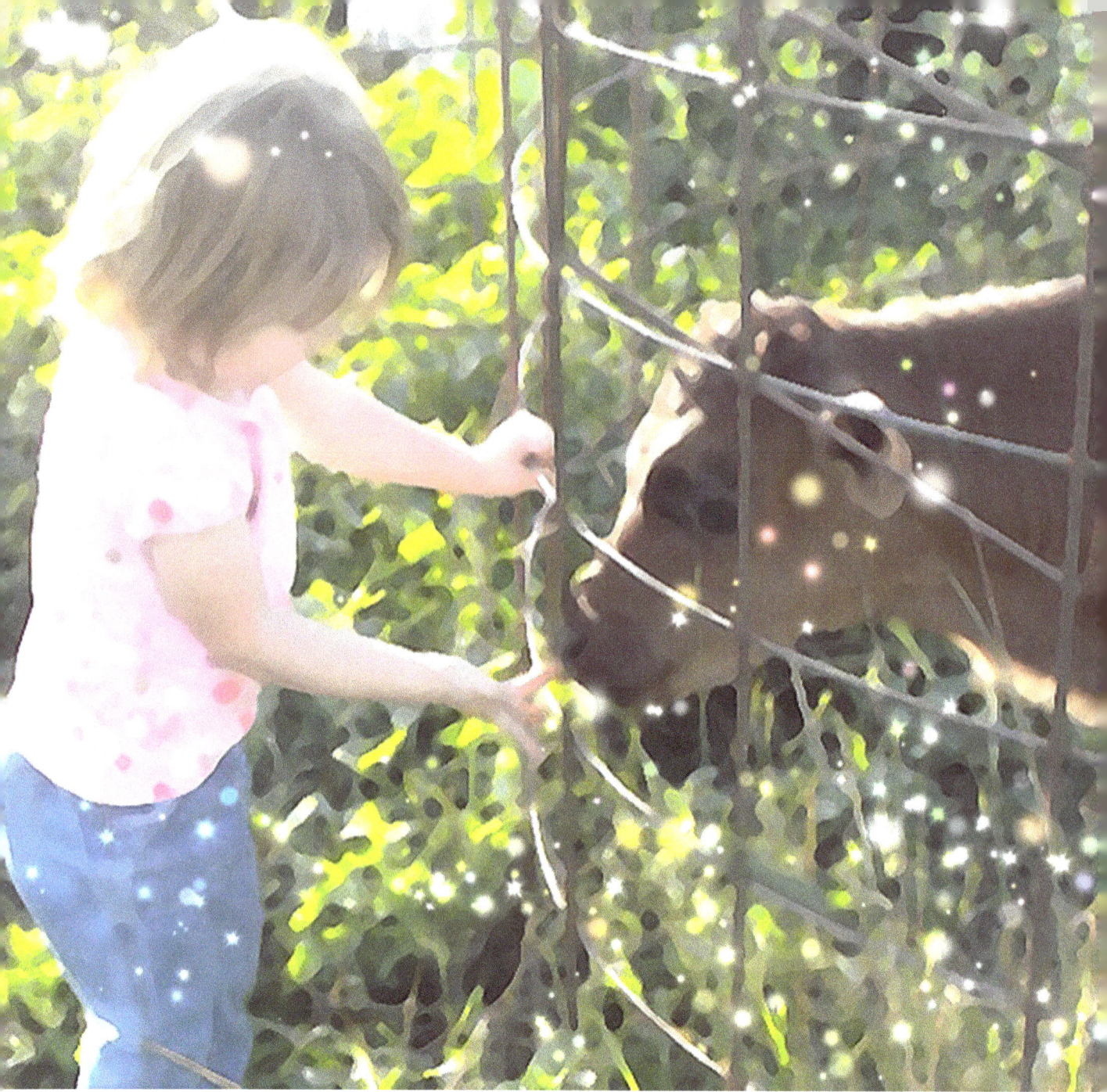

Until then...I have so much to do:
Play tag, hide and seek, and visit the zoo.

I will laugh and run and explore the world,
Eat cake and ice cream that's swirled.

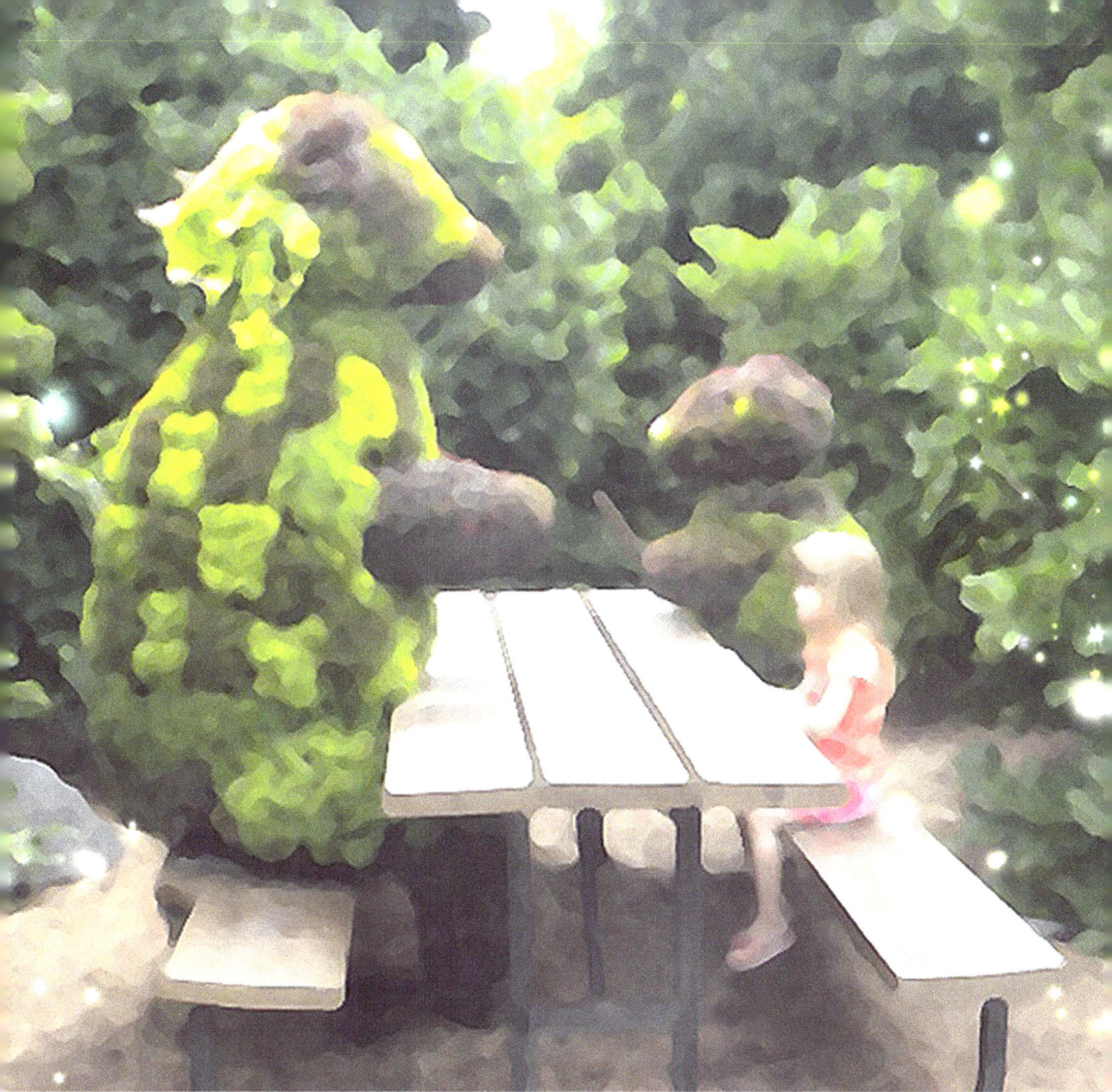

I'll have a picnic, lay back, watch the clouds change shape,
Smell the flowers, soaking up the beautiful landscape.

I give lots of smiles, hugs, and kisses to my family and friends,
Knowing time is so precious and always comes to an end.

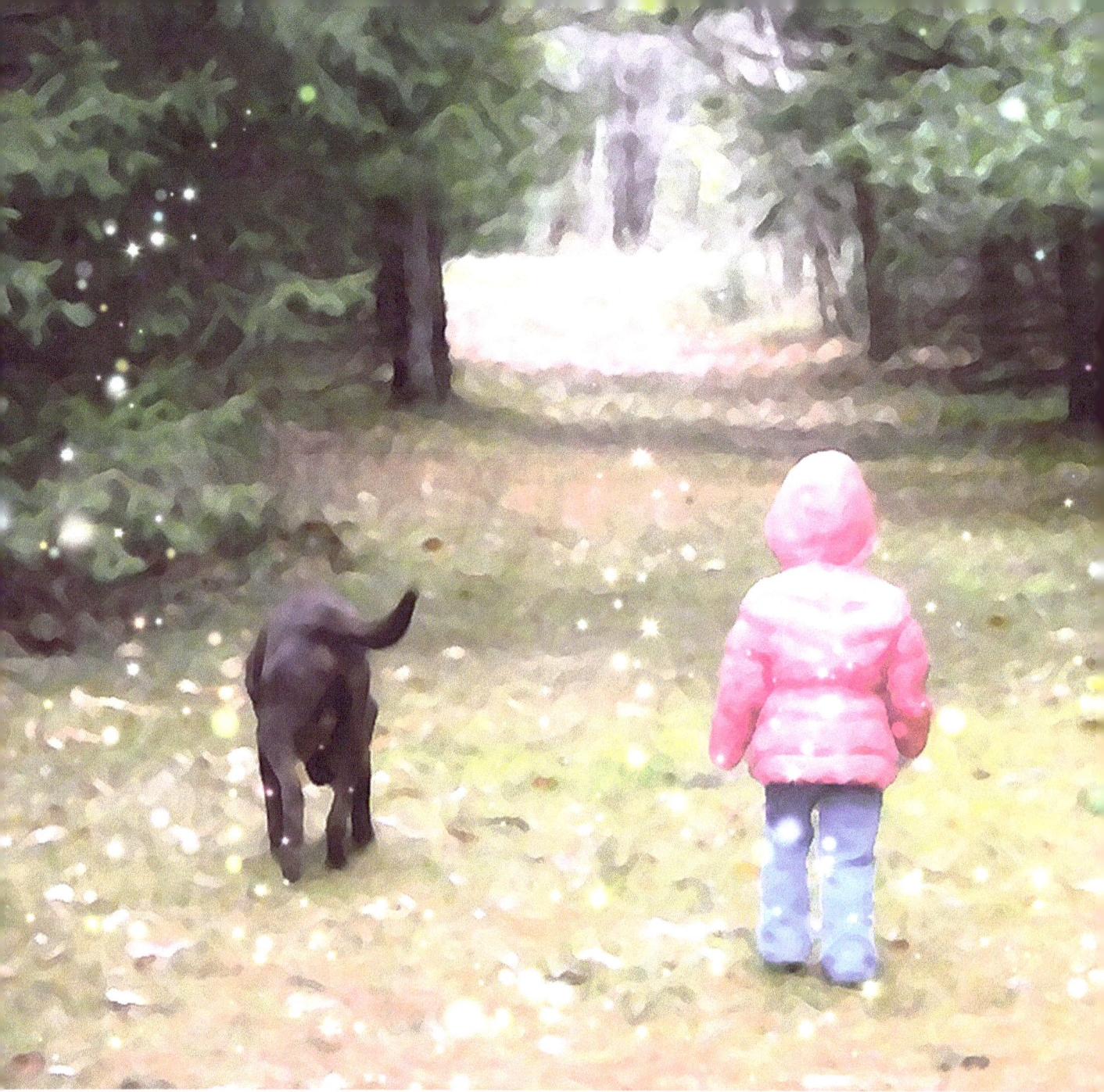

There are many dreams and aspirations for me to achieve.
I can accomplish them all, if I have faith and believe.

First thing's first, I need to stay strong and healthy,
So I follow the advice of my CF posse.

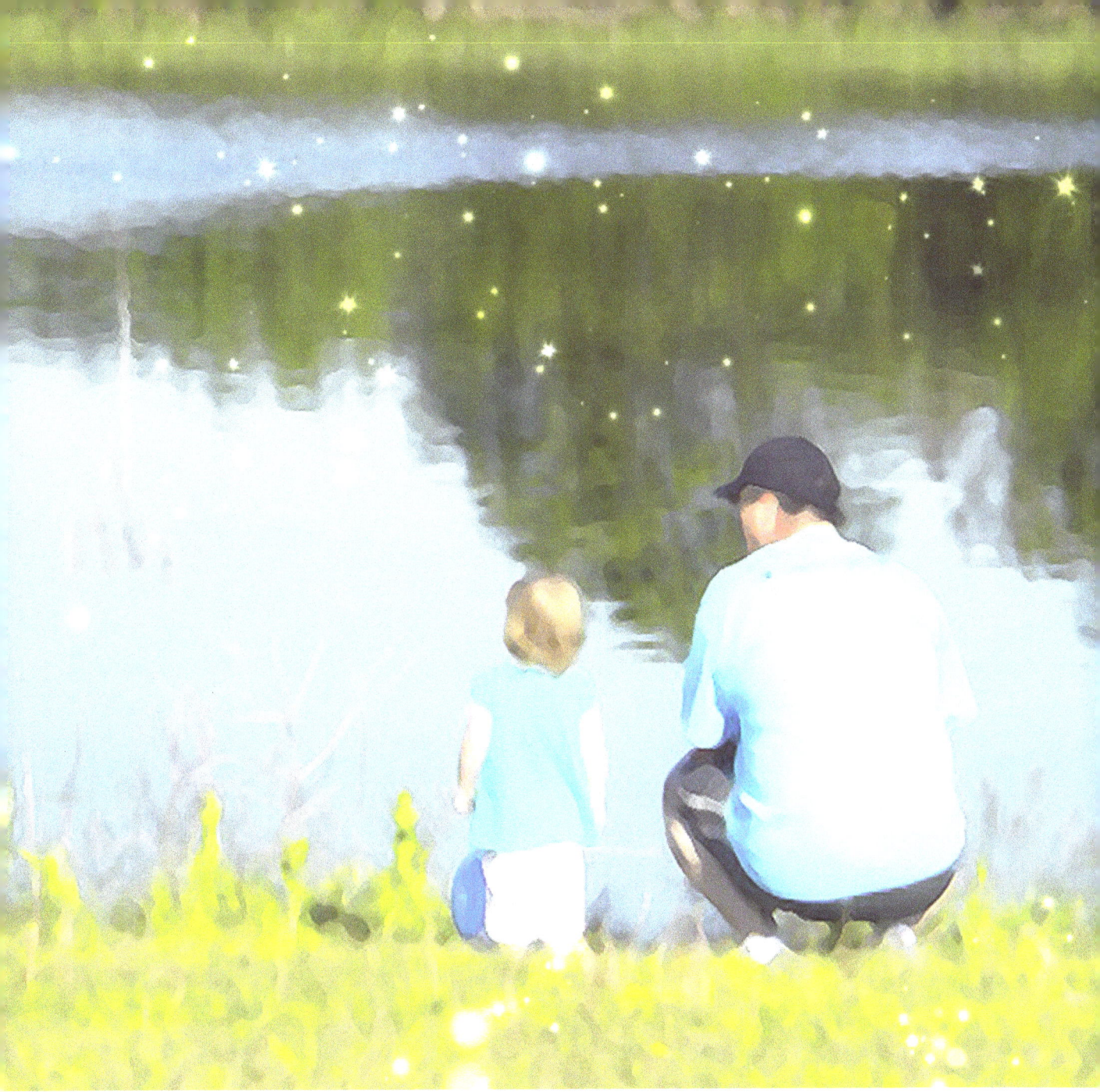

Avoiding smoke and strong fumes is key.
Breathing in those things is hard on me.

We do tapping on my upper body twice a day
On my chest, my back, and my sides, this helps - Hurray!

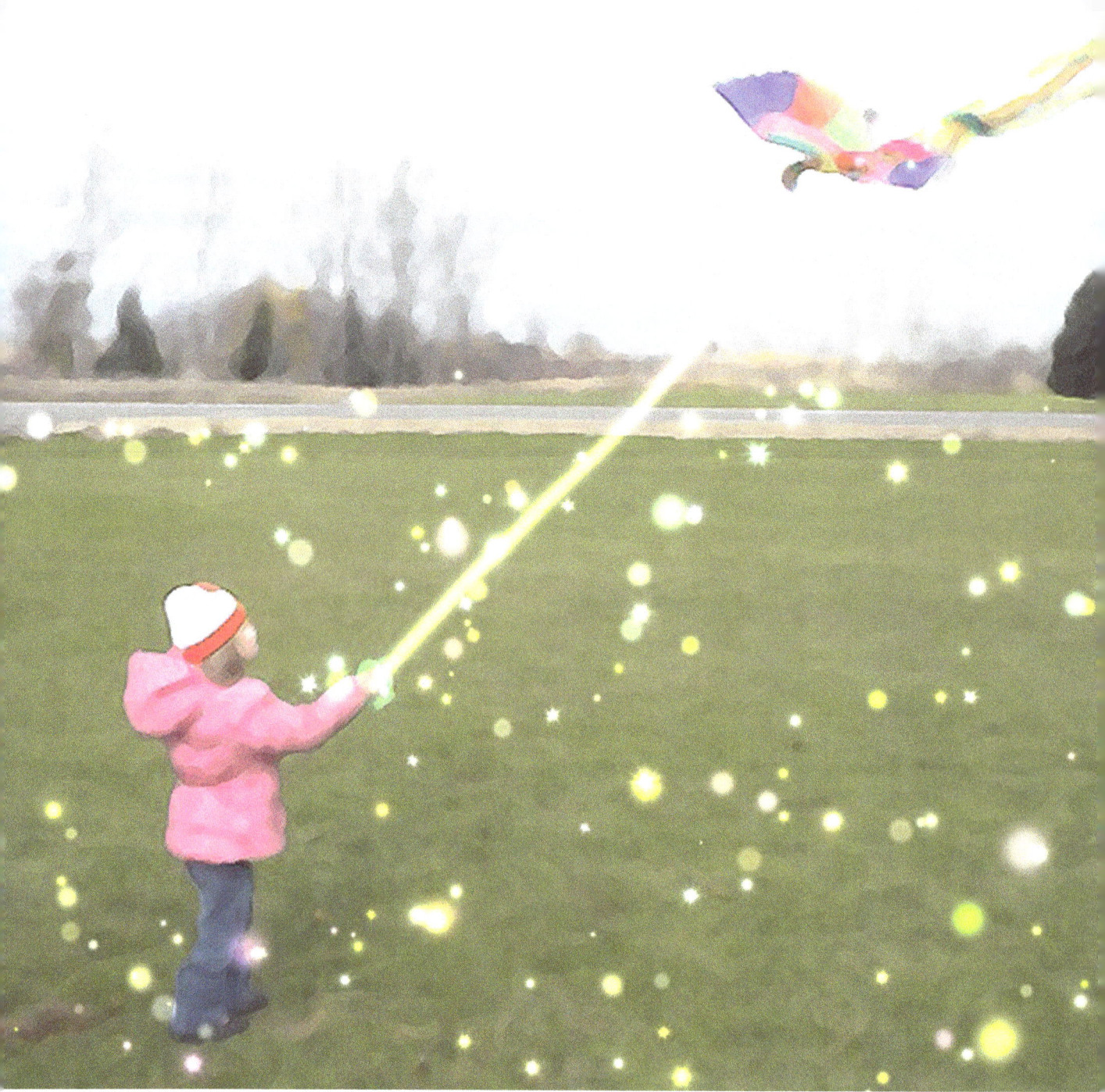

If I get an infection, there are more treatments I have to do:
Extra tapping and inhaling medicine from a nebulizer too.

I take enzymes mixed in applesauce before each meal and snack.
It helps me absorb the proteins and fats in my diet to stay on track.

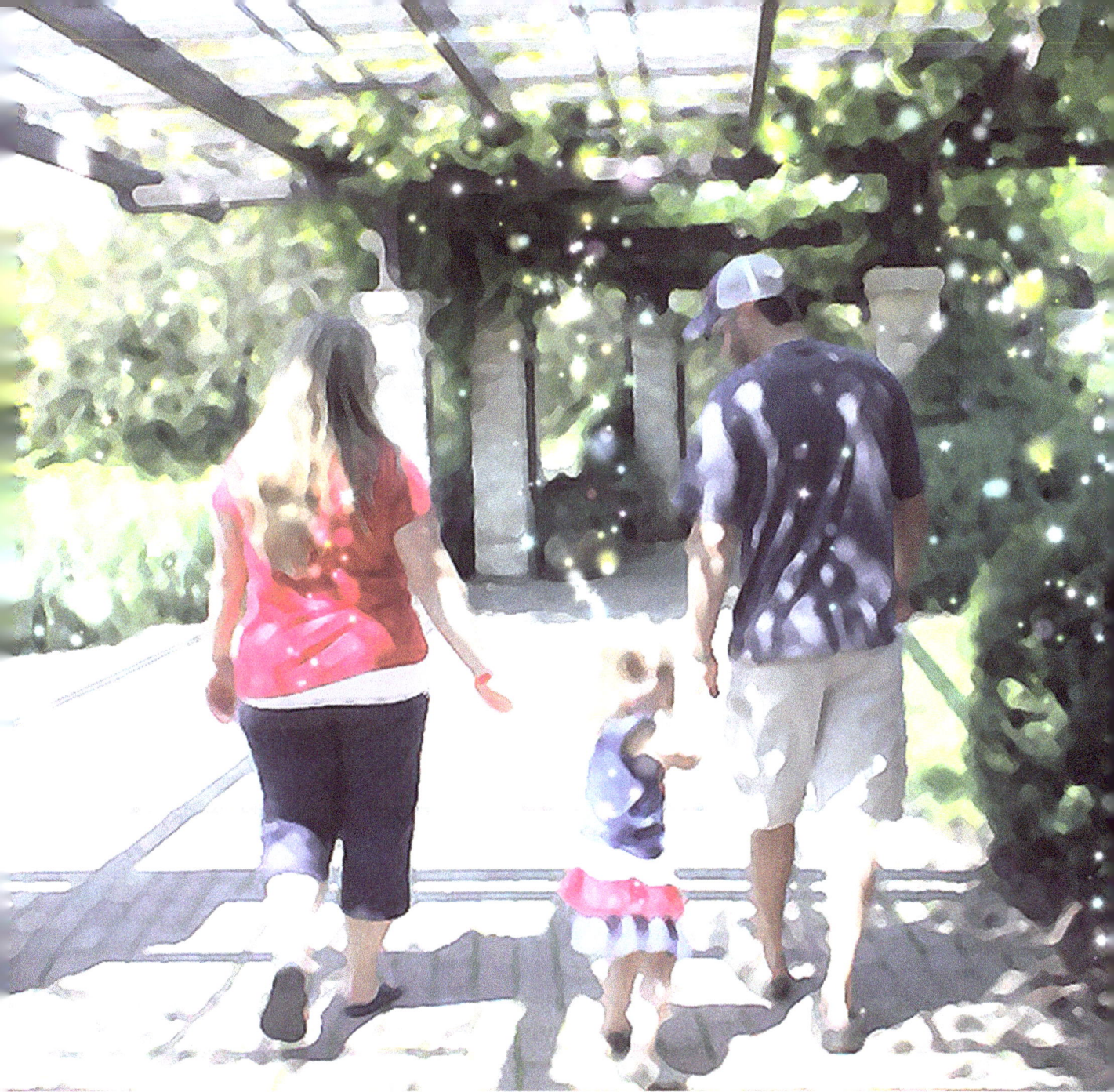

This is really no big deal for me, you see.
I get lots of love and support from my family.

Doing these things prevents trouble in my lungs and tummy,
So I can continue to sing and eat stuff that's yummy.

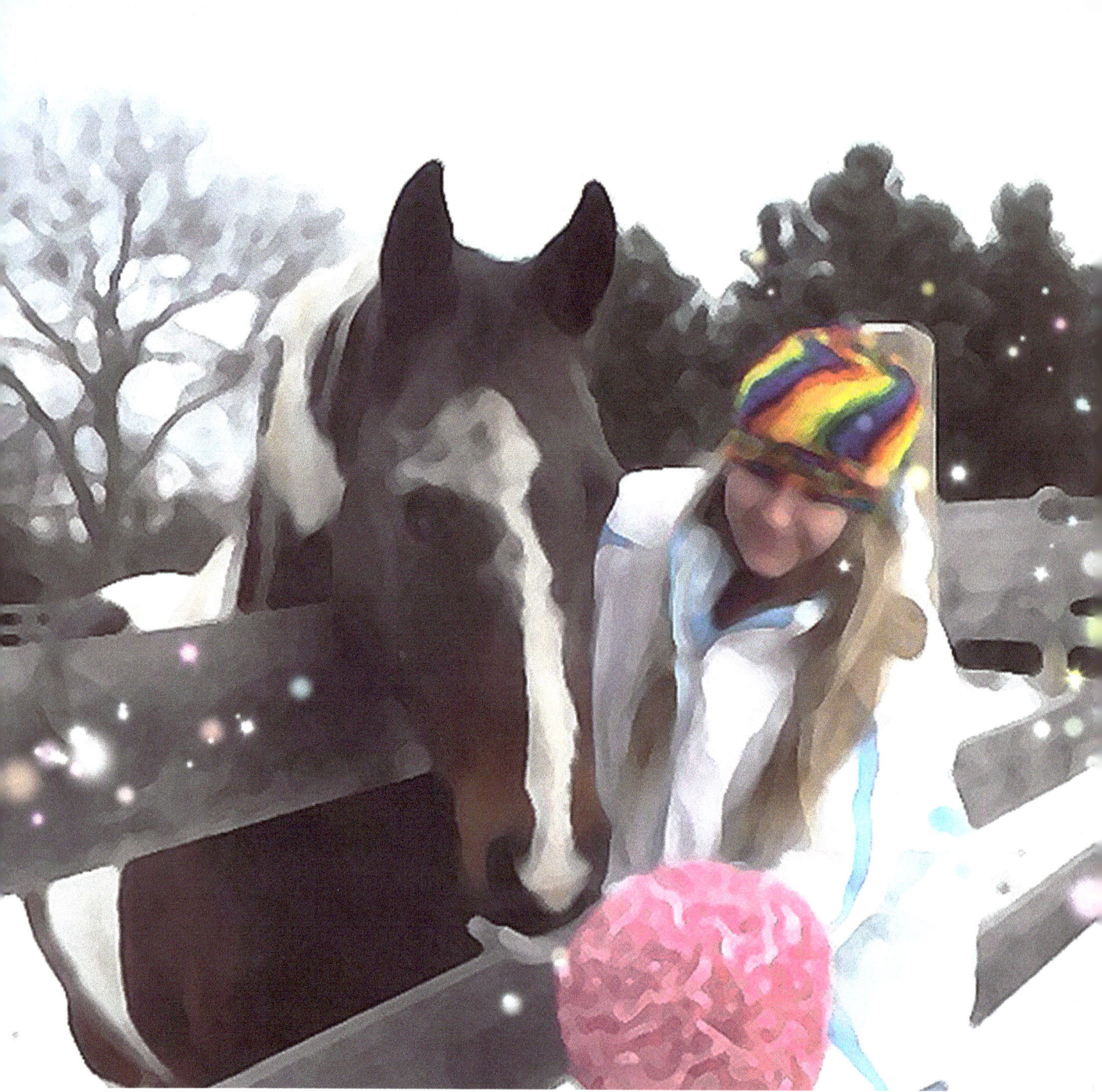

Listening to the experts is in my best interest.
They know what to do to keep me healthiest.

So, mostly I'm the same as the little girls and boys that you know.
I'm just a kid too, who needs a little extra help to grow.

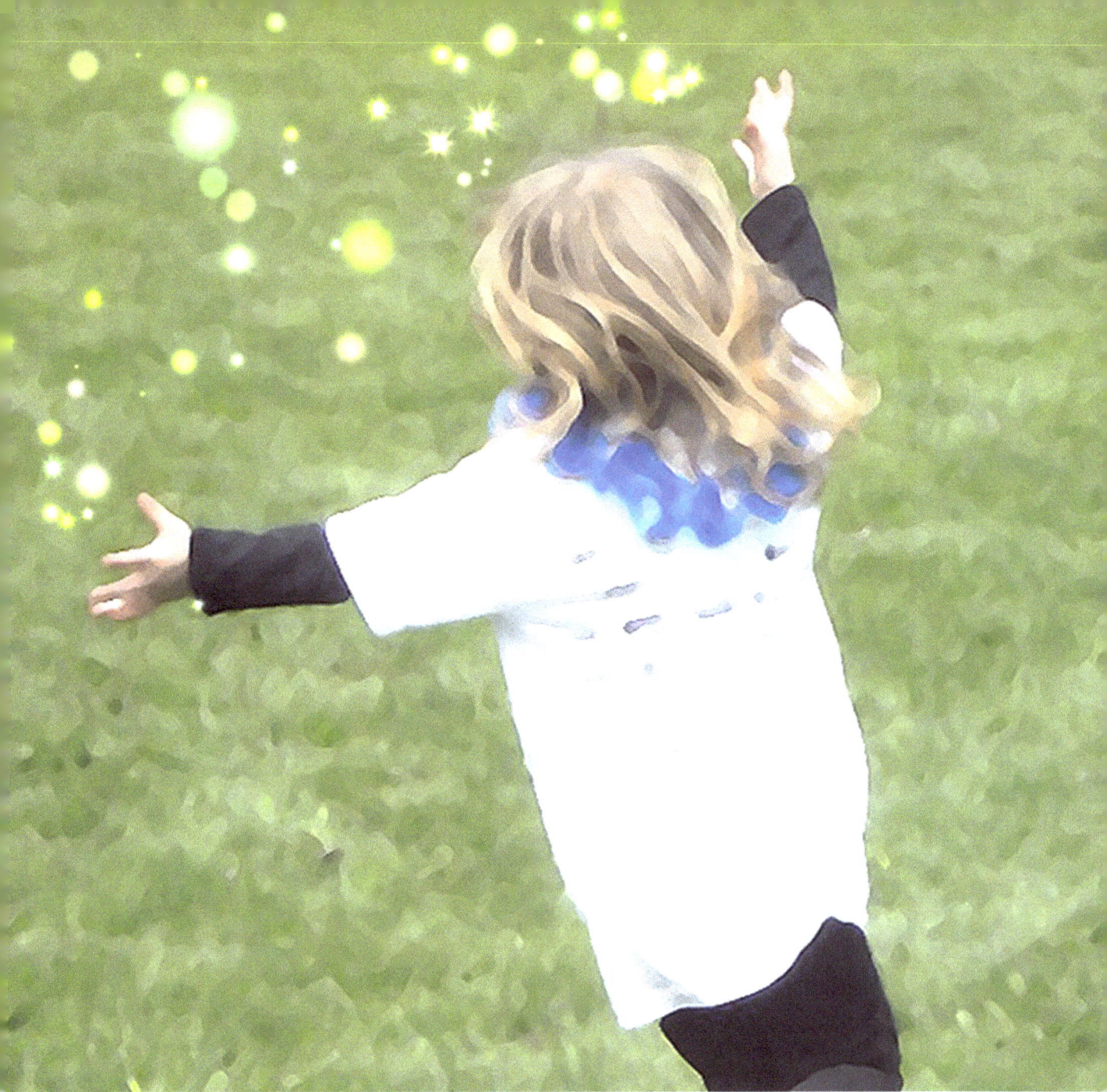

Let's stay positive! There's no reason to be sad or mope.
Believe it! A cure WILL be found, that's what we call:

ALLEGRA'S HOPE

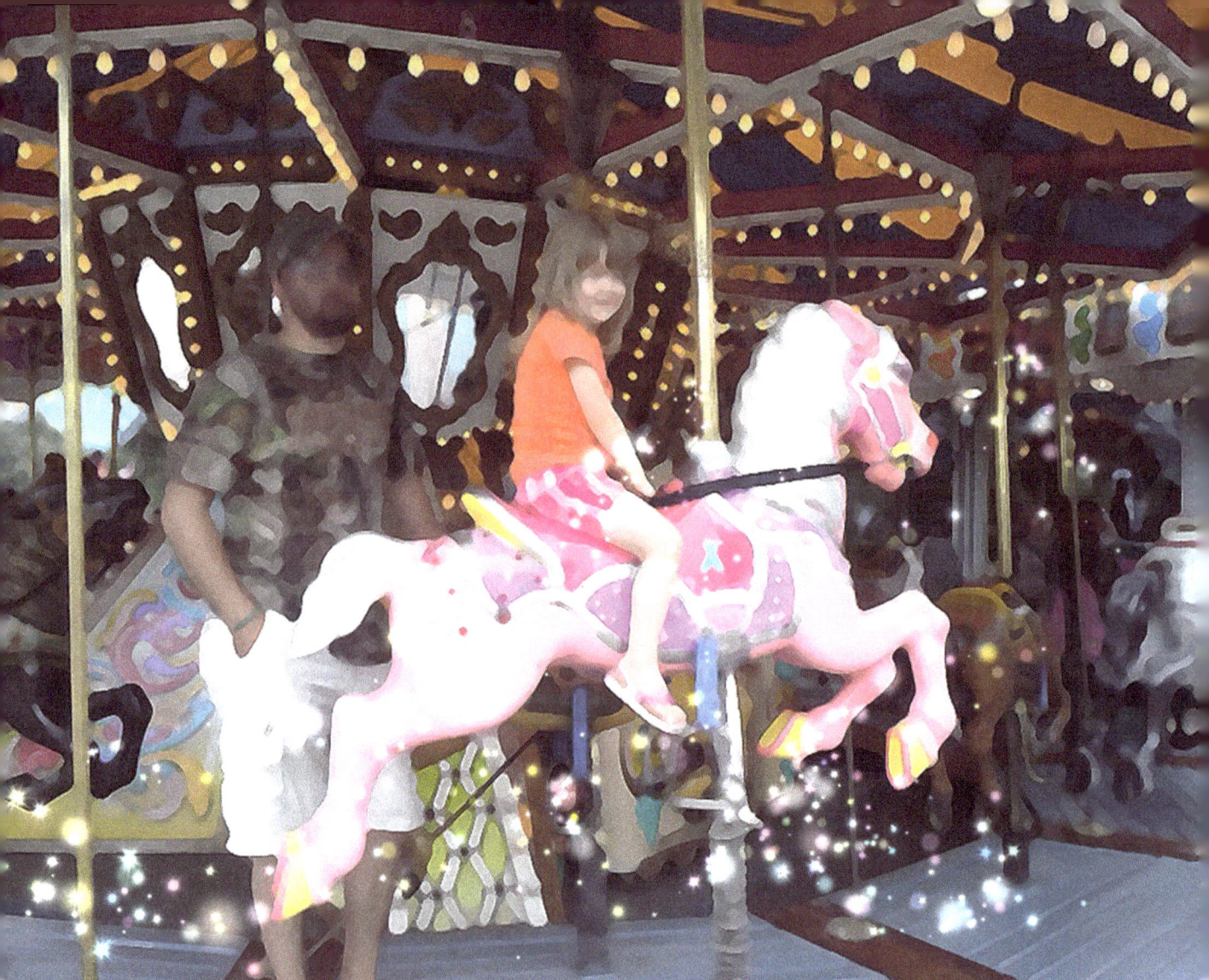

BRIGHT EYES

I love watching you; watching
To see all that you are catching.
You have the most beautiful bright eyes;
So full of confusion, wonder, and surprise.

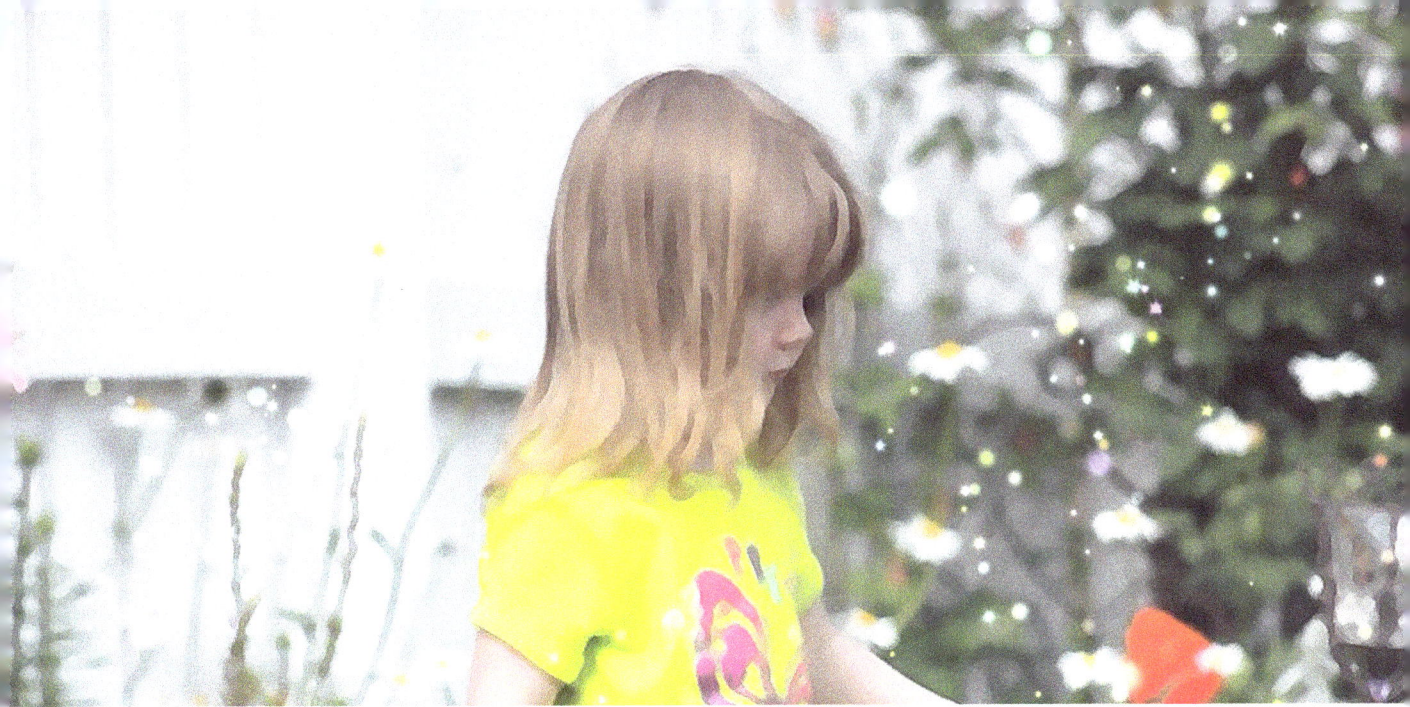

Brand new body, for an old soul.
Those bright eyes like a portal,
Aware and alert, you look.
This lifetime, for you, is a new book.

A multitude of wishes I have for you.
To yourself and your heart always be true.
Allegra, you are perfect exactly as you are.
Dream big and make a wish on every star.

Life is full of lessons to learn.
Let that fire within you burn.
Trust yourself, be strong, be wise.
Only true love for you, Bright Eyes.

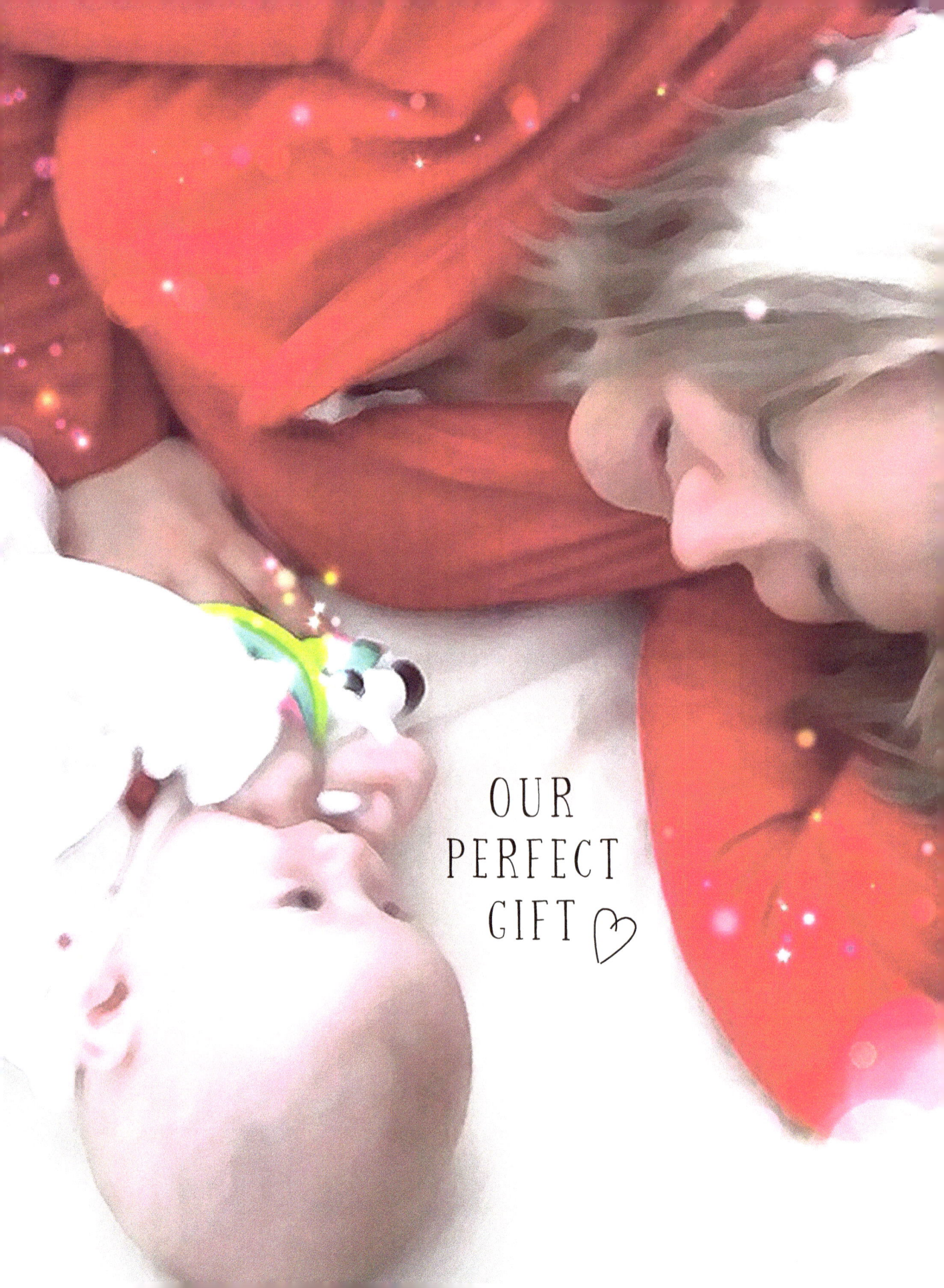

OUR
PERFECT
GIFT ♡

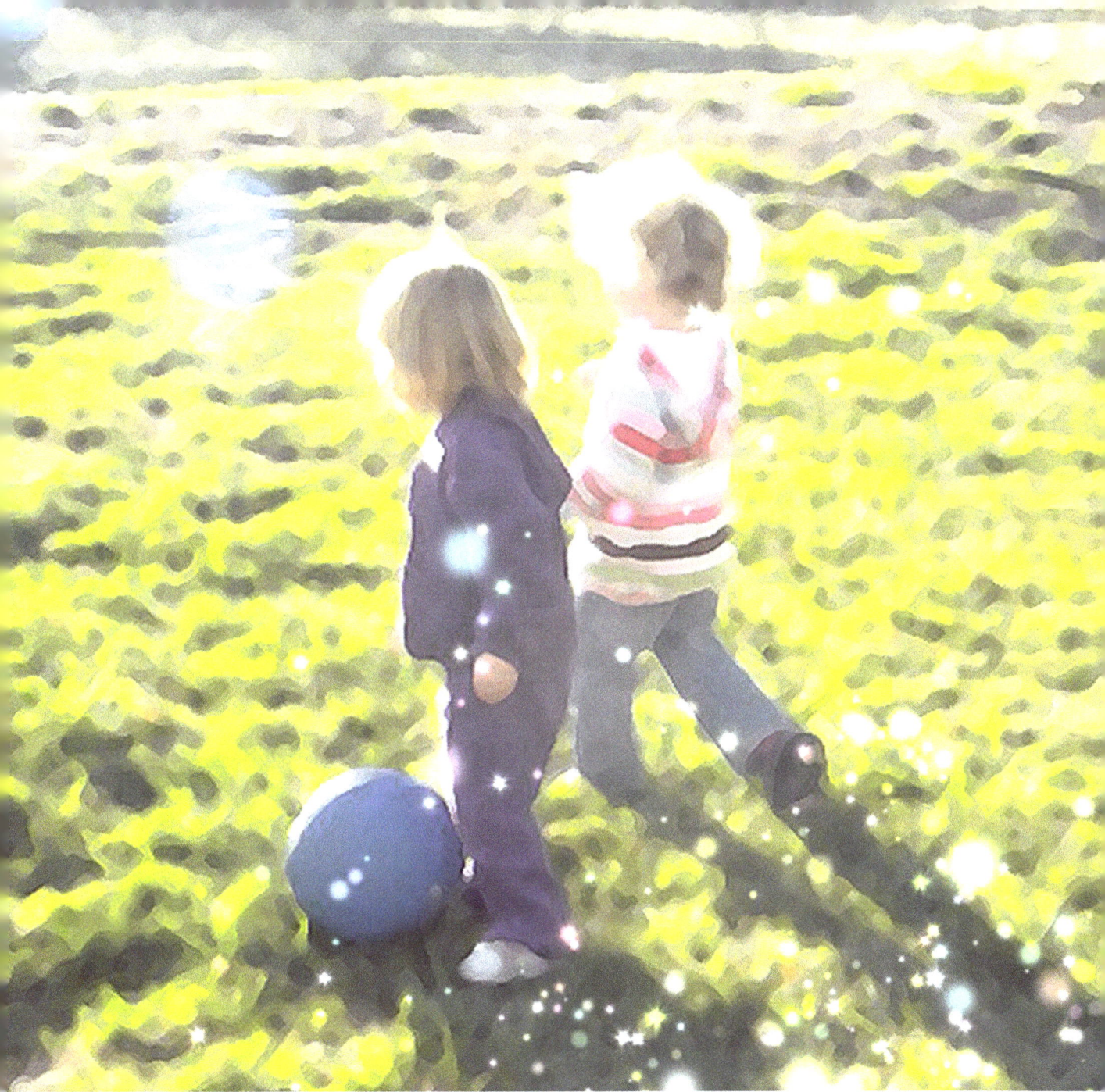

Once upon a magic dream,
Miracles to become the theme,
Sliding down a stray sunbeam,
Fated for us to catch midstream.

Better than rainbows and stars,
Fairies, unicorns, and centaurs,
This gift, the BEST gift by far
Was really supposed to be ours!

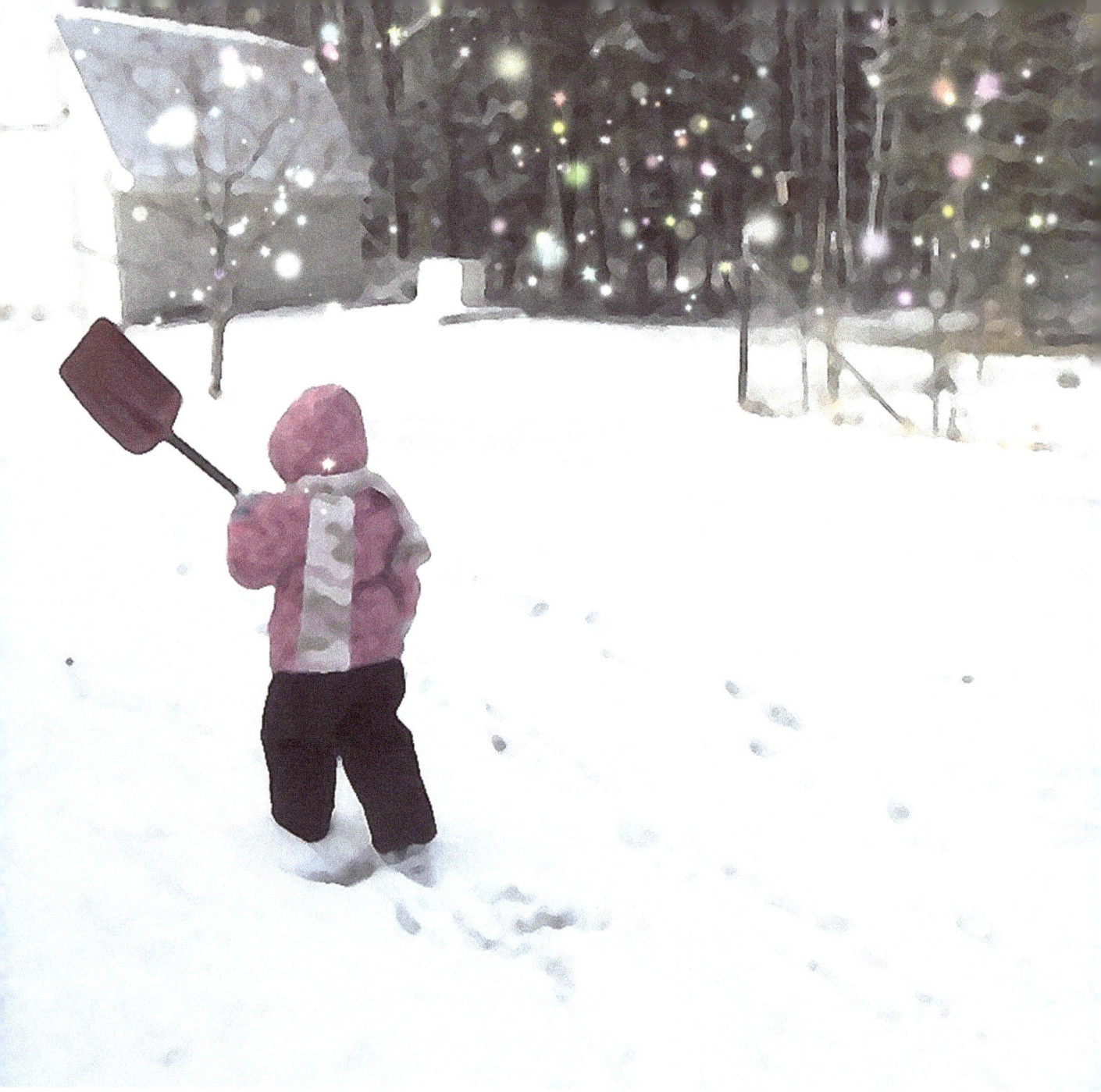

Something we didn't predict,
Unexpected, yet perfect,
As if you were handpicked
The most beautiful prospect.

How could we be so lucky
to become your mommy and daddy?
A blessing and such a sweetie,
you've made us so very happy.

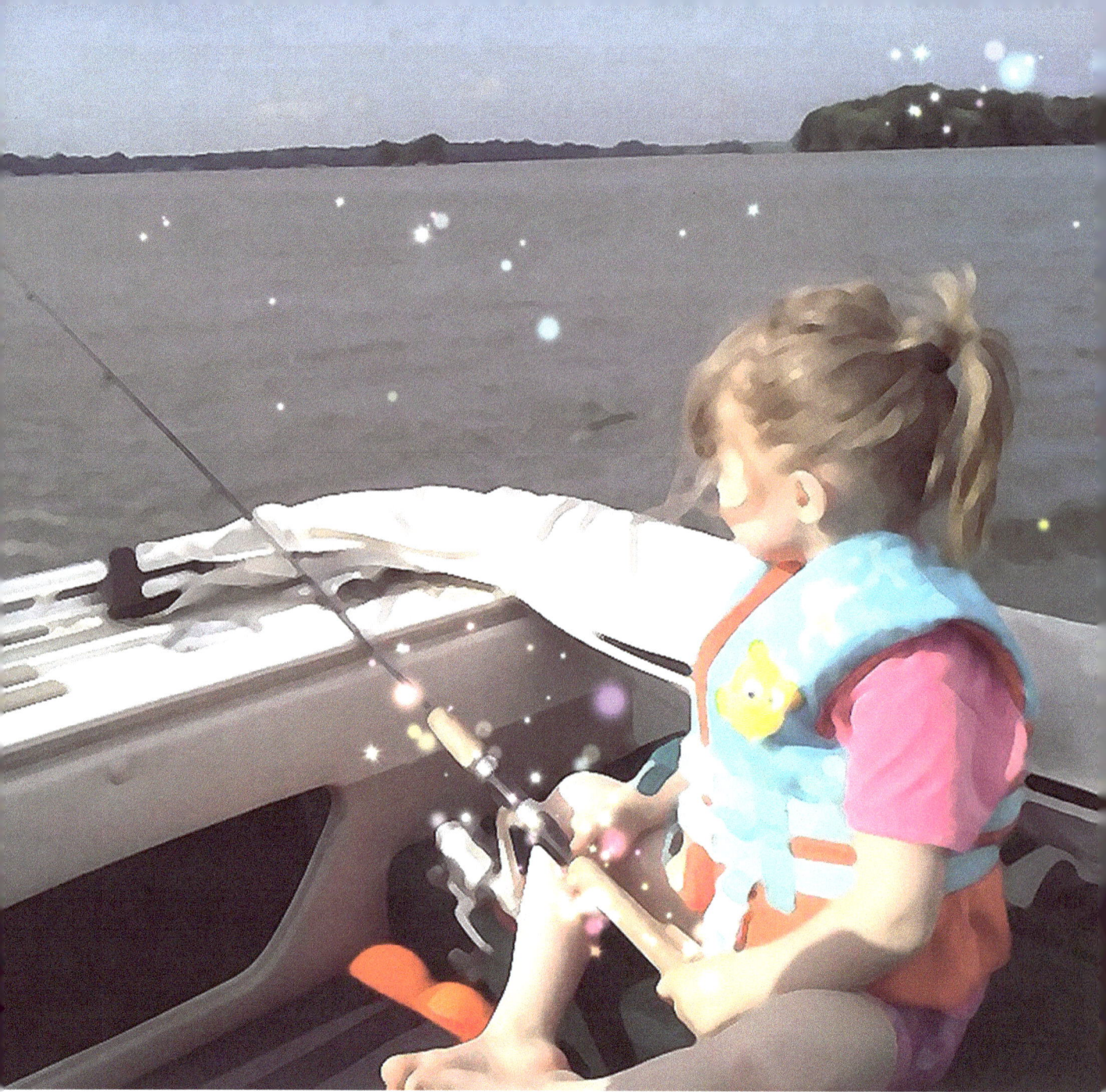

A child is such a pure delight
Like the sun, stars, or moonlight.
But you'll always shine more bright
Than any orb burning day or night.

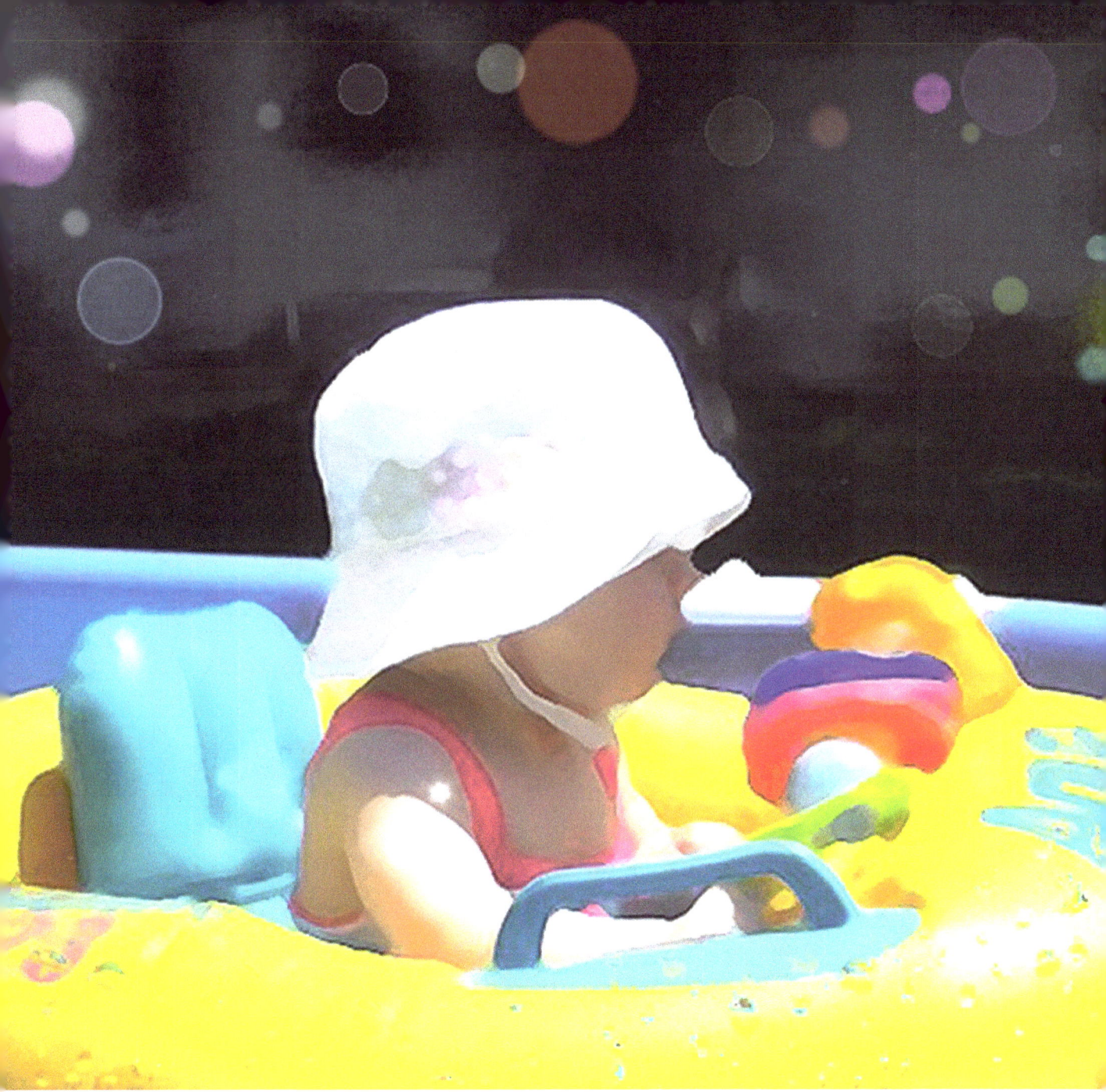

It brings us great pleasure to have you,
Forever we will treasure you
And always hug and kiss you
Daily thanking Heaven for you.

Into our life you came so swift,
Our tiny world made quite a shift!
We're no longer floating adrift,
Anchored by Our Perfect Gift.

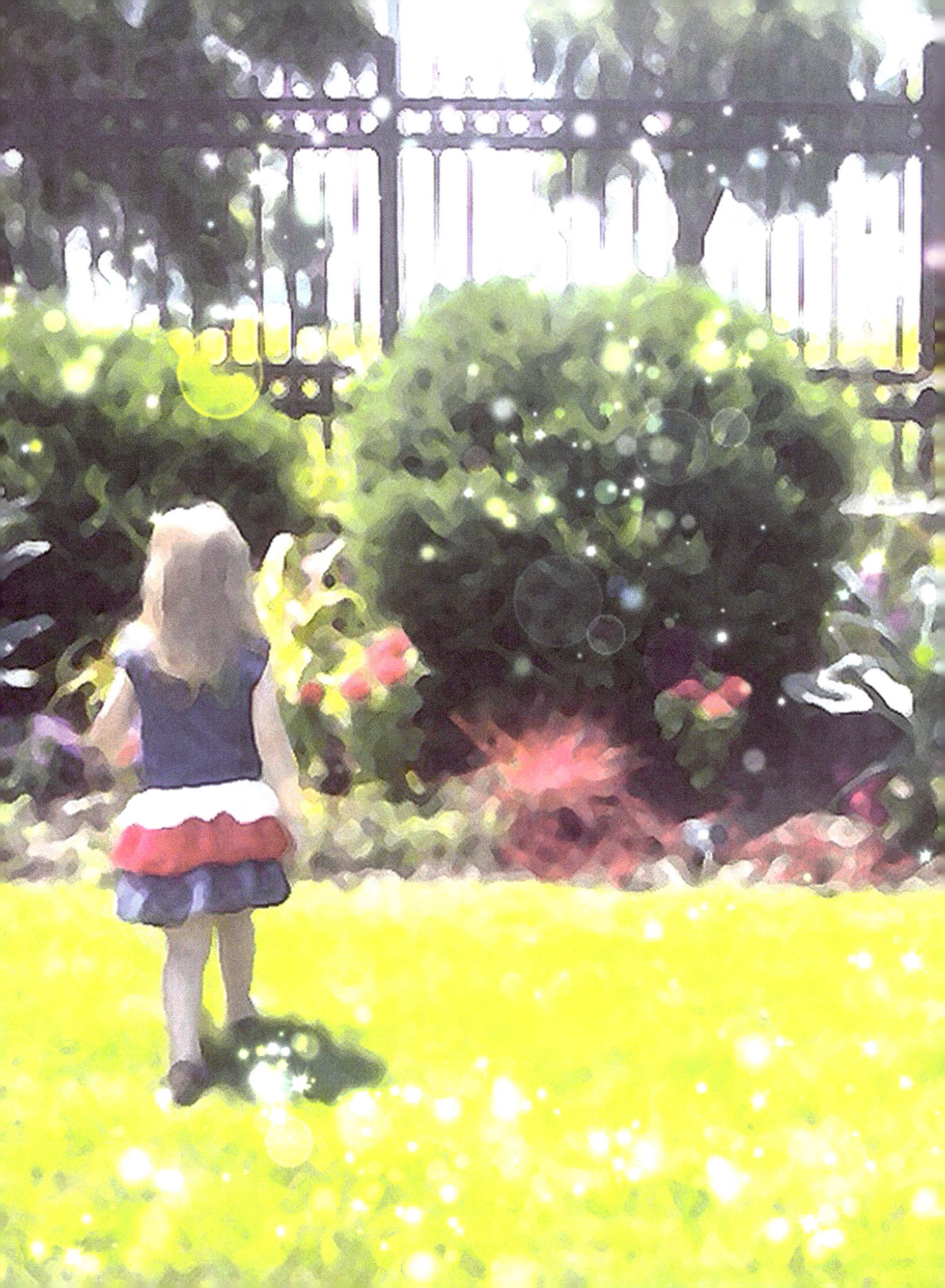

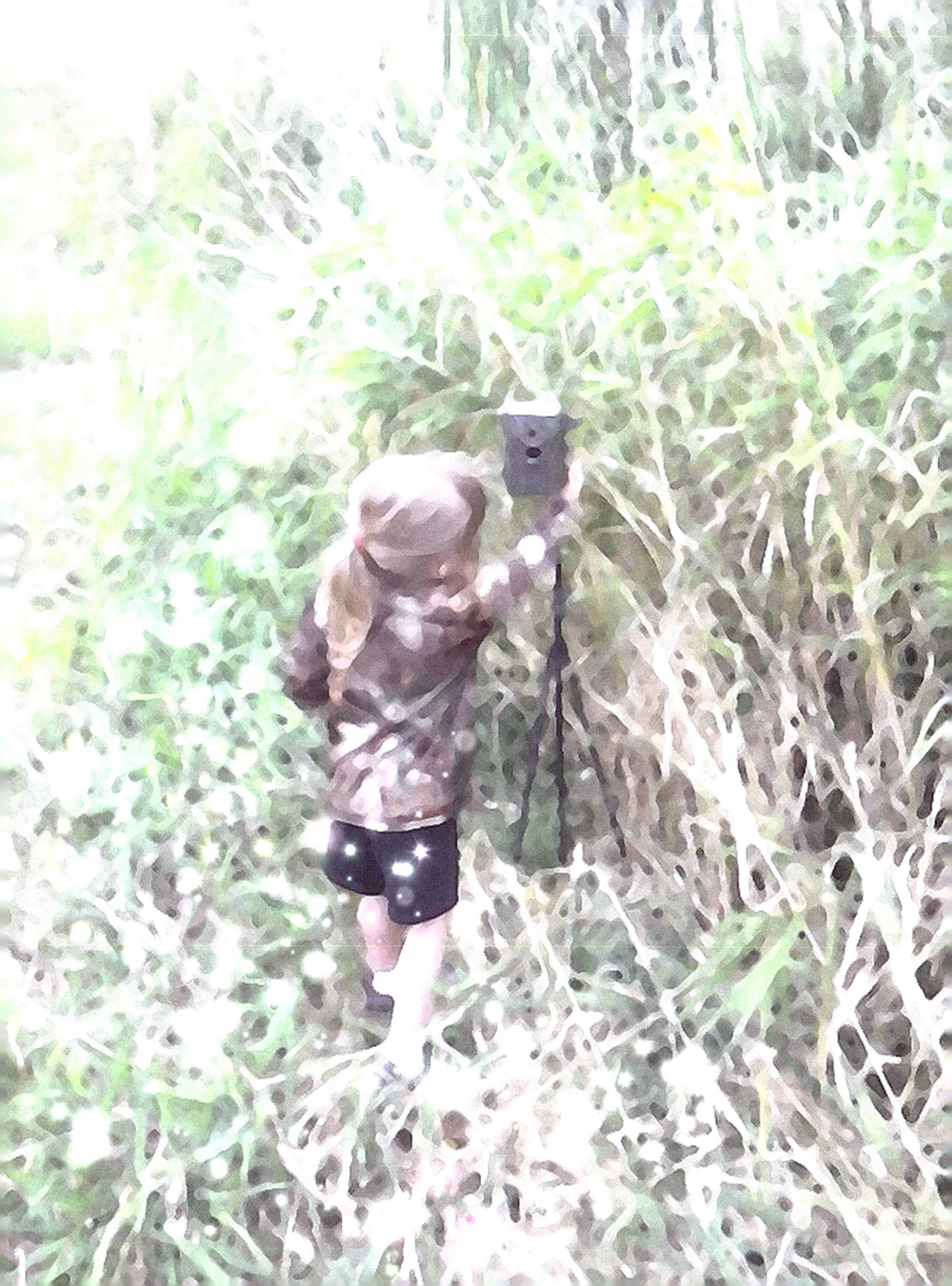

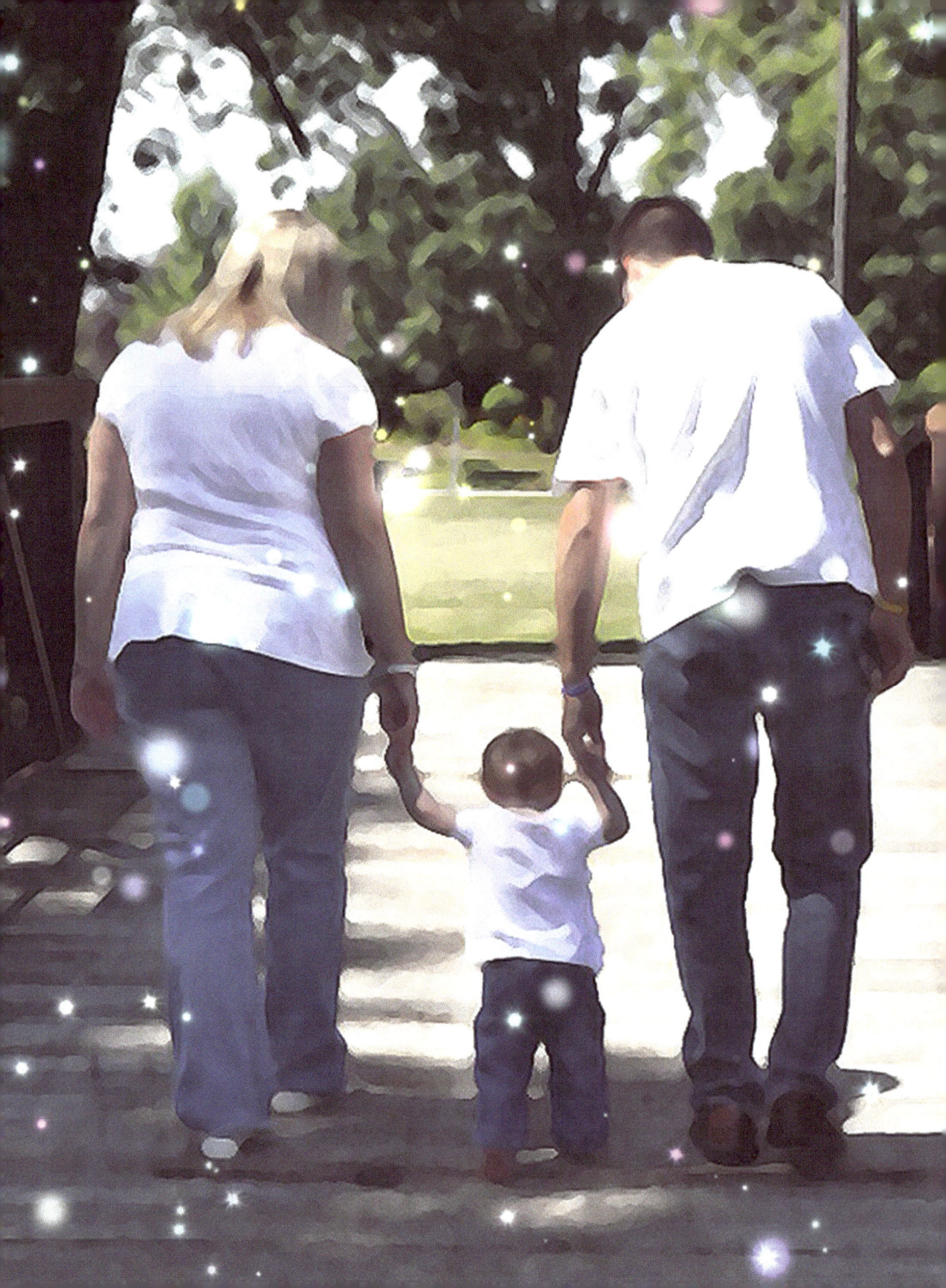

CYSTIC FIBROSIS

On a rainy evening in 2010, we had quite a scare
When our newborn was admitted to intensive care
Obviously this wasn't good, we were quite aware
But for the following news we could not prepare

They told us gently, your daughter has cystic fibrosis
We were in the dark; this was a foreign diagnosis
Regardless of our ignorance, we felt so helpless
Then the real heartbreaker: it's a terminal illness

First we were given the most miraculous present
And then it was being taken back in the next instant
At this moment our faith, hope, and trust were absent
Devastated, heartbroken, the tears we cried were silent

From the beginning, the road wasn't paved smoothly
But wait, this would turn out to be a blessing, truly
Tears were still shed, but it was time to walk bravely
We were now proud parents of a baby girl so lovely

In the days and weeks to come, we sure learned a lot
Along with parenting skills, what to do and what not
There were very special cares that we were to be taught
The way we planned to live had to all be rethought

You see, cystic fibrosis is an inherited chronic disease
It affects the lungs and digestive system, but varies
While some cases are severe, others have fewer worries
All have their treatments for symptoms to try and ease

A guided lifestyle and being proactive are the biggest helpers
Abiding the rules isn't hard, and there isn't much it hampers
As parents we have to be strong and overcome the tempers
Setting a good and consistent example for our little troopers

Doing chest percussions manually or with the vest is a must
Taking enzymes before each snack and meal is an easy adjust
Be very mindful of germs; good hygiene should be focused
It's imperative to avoid any strong fumes, smoke, and dust

For normal growth, they'll have a diet high in calories and fat
I know many people who'd say - wow, you can't beat that!
But good nutrition is linked with better lung function stats
And taking extra vitamins and minerals is a way to combat

It's so important to do all you can to keep them stronger
So life expectancy for these special CFers is much longer
Ultimately it's a cure, the goal for which we are all eager
Please have faith, there is great hope, it's in the near future

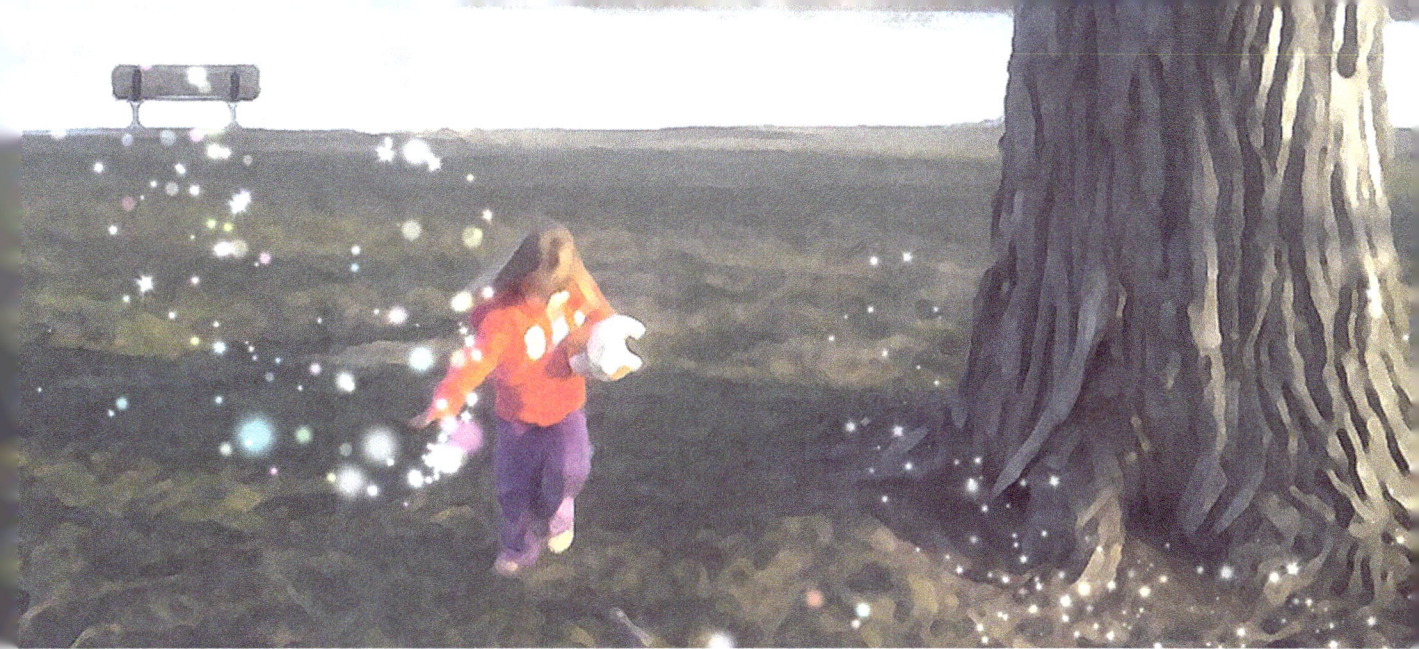

Even though this disease will always leave its unique scar
Advances in research and medical treatment have come far
The possibilities are endless now, and hope is our star
And I believe with all my heart we will win this CF war

All in all, I couldn't be happier with the hand we were dealt
I know so many who've experienced worse than what we felt
Comparatively, we are among the very blessed, I've no doubt
Because of this we've become better people inside and out

This is a case of one door closing and a window opening
The highs always outweigh the lows without questioning
Cystic fibrosis is part of our life, but it's far from defining
Our opportunity to be Allegra's parents makes life worth living

www.ingramcontent.com/pod-product-compliance
Lightning Source LLC
Chambersburg PA
CBHW041611260326
41914CB00012B/1452